Face It With A Puzzle
An OCD WORKBOOK

Volume 2

Face Your Fear
of *Being Imperfect*

By Tammy LaBrake, LCSW-R

INTRODUCTION

OCD has a sneaky way of making people think they ought to be perfect. Does this sound like you:

Somehow you ended up with overly high standards for yourself. You don't hold anyone else to these rules. Why would you? Trying to be perfect isn't an easy way to live. You don't feel good enough, and compliments mean nothing to you.

The life you're living is either too rigid or too chaotic. You wouldn't recommend this way of life to anyone. You're not driven by core values like self-compassion, acceptance or gratitude. Instead, you're motivated by feelings. "I do what I do until it feels just right."

The thought of making a mistake is terrifying. You double triple check your work or avoid it altogether. There's a lot of undoing and redoing. You feel like a reassurance junkie and making a simple decision can be paralyzing at times. If the instructions say, "do this for two minutes" you'll do it for five minutes... just to be sure.

Sometimes you put things off because you know that striving for perfection takes all the fun away. There is a lot of procrastination. Waiting until the last possible moment to get something done allows you to say, "I was in a hurry." It's not an accurate reflection of your capabilities because you were rushed.

You put things off, or spend too much time on a task. It doesn't have to be like this. You have every right to be hopeful and live a carefree life. But, first you must learn to tolerate feeling "just wrong." Learn to love all your imperfections.

Perfection is the Enemy of Growth

Seeking perfection is an unattainable goal and leads to a life not lived.

Striving for perfection is the same thing as trying for certainty. That's how OCD gets a hold of you. If you believe perfection is possible, then OCD will gladly give you all kinds of ideas on how to try and achieve it.

OCD isn't just the doubting disease. It's the anti-doubting disease. You have a brain that is against doubt and uncertainty. Your mind is hyper-focused on achieving certainty and perfectionism is just another way of trying to get it.

Learning how to be "just wrong" will help you break free from living such a rigid, hard life. If you have a growth mindset, mistakes are nothing but opportunities to learn.

Perfection is the enemy of growth. Notice your imperfections and say, "Good, I'm still a growing human being." You'll find freedom in a growth mindset and imprisonment in a perfection mindset. In fact, you'll probably find mistakes in this Workbook. *Message from the author: I'd rather make mistakes than never complete the project. Email me (tammy@bossitback.com) when you find my mistakes so that I can feel the anxiety, allow the discomfort, tolerate it and celebrate being productively imperfect.*

Exposure and Response Prevention (ERP)

ERP is a therapy that uses gradual or systematic desensitization to help people with OCD overcome fears. This type of therapy encourages you to engage in activities that purposefully create anxiety and doubt. When you do these exercises, you provoke the anxiety but do nothing to relieve the discomfort.

Since you may not be ready yet to throw caution to the wind and live an imperfect carefree life, this workbook offers a milder way to become desensitized to being imperfect or feeling "just wrong."

How to Use the Puzzles

These puzzles are made with words and phrases often associated with being imperfect. Some of the words reflect how uncomfortable it feels to feel "just wrong." How you react to the discomfort is the key. Lean into it, not away from it.

Other puzzles have more to do with the consequences of trying to be perfect or feel "just right." You always have a choice to feed or starve OCD. Not that saying no to OCD is easy but if you decide to feed OCD, at least do it mindfully and recognize what it will cost you to obey OCD. So some of these puzzles will help you to think twice about the cost of trying to be perfect.

You might be so focused on solving the puzzle that you experience no anxiety until the puzzle is solved and you suddenly realize the phrase or words are uncomfortable. So your anxiety might get triggered while you're solving a puzzle, or not until after the puzzle is solved and you realize what it says.

Words and phrases are repeated several times in this workbook. When using ERP as a treatment modality, repetition is essential. You need to repeat the same exposures over and over until they have little to no effect.

Repetition breeds boredom. Your brain gets bored doing the same exposure over and over. A common mistake people make when doing ERP is that they don't do an exposure enough. So these puzzles repeatedly expose you to possible trigger words associated with being imperfect.

Hope with all your might that these puzzles trigger your anxiety. Intentionally triggering your anxiety is a good thing! Because when your anxiety is triggered, you get to practice your skills. You get good at what you practice. Practice makes... I hope you didn't just say perfect! Practice makes progress!

Not all of the puzzles will be anxiety producing. Some of them just help you practice the best way to talk to OCD. When talking to OCD, it's important to say as little as possible. Don't explain or rationalize. Don't try to use logic. Just get to the shrug as quickly as possible.

"Eh, whatever." ¯_(ツ)_/¯

How to Use the Exposure Worksheets

In addition to the puzzles, there are worksheets to help you create even more discomfort. Finding opportunities to bring on your anxiety is one of the fiercest ways to manage OCD. Resisting compulsions while creating anxiety is like Kryptonite to OCD. It deprives OCD of its powers. It's hard to be anxious when you want to be anxious.

The exposure worksheets consist of repeatedly writing anxiety-provoking words, telling a story or using stick figures to draw out your worst case scenario. Rate your anxiety at the beginning and end of each worksheet. Continue the exercise until your anxiety drops. Use additional sheets of paper if needed.

If used repeatedly and without any compulsive responses, these worksheets can help you defy OCD. If a particular word or phrase is overwhelming, then write it out on the worksheet as many times as it takes to become desensitized. Be sure to include any troublesome words of your own that you don't find in any of the puzzles.

If you like to sketch, use the worksheets to draw scenes of situations that tend to make you feel imperfect. You don't have to be an artist to draw. Using stick figures draw four scenes playing out your worst fear. In the first scene, you have realized you can never be perfect or feel "just right." And then what happens next? What might happen because you're imperfect? Draw that.

And then what happens? Draw that. In the final scene, draw the worst unhappy ending you can imagine as a result of being imperfect and feeling "just wrong."

While you are drawing or writing words, if you notice any anxiety, say: "Good there's my anxiety. I want this. I need the practice." Repeat what you are drawing or writing as many times needed to become desensitized.

Remember, when you're triggered, it's crucial to practice accepting the anxiety and agreeing with the worry. Don't try to prove OCD wrong or right. Just say, "Yup, that could happen. It would be unpleasant but not dangerous."

A Special Message From the Author: The Worksheets might not seem as rewarding as the puzzles. They are equally as important and the repetition is necessary. To make it worth your effort send me (Tammy) an email of how you used the Worksheets. Send me pictures if you like. I will return an email to you with a secret code giving you access to one of my hidden blog posts at blog.bossitback.com.

If you complete your Worksheets you should get a reward! Email me about your Worksheets and I'll send you the secret code. You'll be pleasantly surprised! Email: tammy@bossitback.com

Healthy Bonus

Some of the puzzles are more difficult than others to solve. That's because there is a second purpose of this workbook. It takes dopamine to defy OCD. When you persevere and work on solving the puzzles you will produce dopamine--a neurotransmitter that provides fuel for ongoing motivation.

OCD is a big force to go up against, so you need motivation and determination to persevere. Never quit. The day you quit is the day you were going to win.

So not only do these puzzles act as an exposure exercise, and teach you how to talk to OCD, but because they are puzzles they activate healthy logical parts of your brain. It's much harder for OCD to influence you when all parts of your brain are activated. Solving puzzles can make your brain a lean, mean, fighting machine.

Some of the puzzles are tough to solve. There are clues sprinkled throughout the book for the more difficult puzzles but use the hints sparingly. Challenge your brain as much as possible!

Now that you know how to use this workbook, it's time to Face It With a Puzzle!

THE COST OF PERFECTIONISM

T HE NEED to feel "just right" is costing you. Feeling "just right" isn't worth it. Think about what you're being robbed of while trying to feel "just right."

What are you giving up to feel "just right" or avoid mistakes? Are your relationships affected? Are you less productive? Do you beat yourself up and lack self-compassion? Have you lost confidence in yourself? Are you losing sleep?

Write down what it's costing you to seek perfection and feel "just right."

THE BENEFITS OF
BEING PERFECTLY IMPERFECT

NOW THAT YOU'VE ACKNOWLEDGED what seeking perfection is costing you, let's look at what you're fighting for.

If you stop seeking perfection and accept feeling "just wrong" what do you gain? How would your life improve? What would life be like to surrender to mistakes and imperfections?

Anybody who claims to be perfect or feel "just right" all the time, has stopped growing as a person. We are meant to be imperfect and uncertain. If you can see your imperfections as normal and acceptable, write down how that will improve the quality of your life.

You've got to care about something deeper than feeling "just right." What is it that you care more about? Write down why you're fighting this fight.

The following words can be found in the diagram below reading forward, backward, up, down and diagonally. Find the words and circle them.

wrong
wrinkled
endless
overrun
useless
messy

tardy
inept
tears

U N U R R E V O L H F A H V R T

G S U G C O Z Z L A Z U W P H E

J J E X X B O Y J A T A R D Y A

F K M L M P M U L D B F O J E R

U I I N E P T E G I D A N Y K S

K H H H J S V F S W K C G I X R

U S C X U I S H Z D P D J Y H J

W S T E A B N W G F S R H B P Z

W I C U C K B B N R F W P M G M

E Z Q E B D A H S I T Z Q U P Q

R X S L Z C N B Q S E G N U S T

G X T W B U A Y S S E M C C J V

B Z Q R Q H O I T O L L G P B K

W P F O I L M B I N W I D Q Y R

L A R C R H K F Q D T B K N J D

D E L K N I R W V F S A U B E M

Puzzle 1

Each of these Cryptograms is a message in substitution code. THE SILLY DOG might become UJD WQPPZ BVN if U is substituted for T, J for H, D for E, etc. One way to break the code is to look for repeated letters. E, T, A, O, N, R and I are the most often used letters. A single letter is usually A or I; OF, IS and IT are common 2-letter words; try THE or AND for a 3-letter group. The code is different for each Cryptogram.

1. Ds dw gfus ds dw uvj D urrpms sfdw
_I _a _e _h
ypptdvo by jbba. (Clue:It's all about acceptance.)
_d

2. L icmn L bcrn vj kdxlt cw kicfzik
_I _s _t _o
xts bccp wccblri.
(Clue: I'd rather look scatterbrained than worry about looking scatterbrained.)

3. Hdnhgd flgg sdcdcyds cd qns ck
_P _l _m
lchdsqdxzlniv. (This will be on my gravestone: She wasn't perfect.)
_o

More Tips: First try to figure out the vowels. Consider if double letters in the middle of a word could be vowels. Other two letter words include: to, do, be, my, me.

WORKSHEET

Use this worksheet to write anxiety-provoking, troublesome words. Fill the page with words that trigger your anxiety about being imperfect. You are uncomfortable. There is a strong urge to "make it right." What does imperfect feel like? If there are words associated with being imperfect, gross or "just wrong" that trigger your anxiety, write those words down here, repeatedly. Fill up the page. Note your anxiety level (on a scale of 0-100) at the beginning and end of this exercise.

Anxiety level at start __

Anxiety level at end ___ (If your anxiety hasn't dropped, repeat this Worksheet.)

Each of these Cryptograms is a message in substitution code. THE SILLY DOG might become UJD WQPPZ BVN if U is substituted for T, J for H, D for E, etc. One way to break the code is to look for repeated letters. E, T, A, O, N, R and I are the most often used letters. A single letter is usually A or I; OF, IS and IT are common 2-letter words; try THE or AND for a 3-letter group. The code is different for each Cryptogram.

1. Q'ť izqvi až tbxy agqě tqeabxy b̌vl
bkkzs agy b̌voqyah az zuymsgykt tў.

(Clue: Experience anxiety as an unpleasant sensation.)

2. P box̌uoghjiq zjq̌lfǒh up̌jwf.

3. G tědzcx wup̌okfť m̌fgepk.

Clue: Failure doesn't exist.
Watch Koby Bryant's YouTube video on failure, "What Drives Winning."

Tammy (the author) has purposefully allowed errors in this book for all the world to see. Her poor craftsmanship will surely bring criticism and disapproval. Oh well...

Puzzle 3

To solve this puzzle, fill in the blanks below with the correct missing letter and then transfer the letter to the corresponding numbered square in the diagram below. Be careful! The puzzle is not as simple as it may first appear!

1.	2.	3.	4.	5.	6.	7.

1. f a _ l t y

2. t e a r _

3. w _ a k

4. a w f u _

5. m _ s s y

6. c h a o _

7. _ l o w

Puzzle 4

WORKSHEET

Use this worksheet to repeatedly write any troublesome words. Add your own anxiety-provoking words. Fill the page with words that trigger your anxiety about never feeling "just right." What would it feel like if you kept making mistakes or bad decisions? Write these words repeatedly. Let the anxiety rise and just notice it. Don't judge the anxiety as good or bad.

Anxiety level at start __

Anxiety level at end ___

The spaces between the words in the following message has been eliminated and divided into pieces. Rearrange the pieces to reconstruct the messages. The dashes indicate the number of letters in each word.

EILO DLOO KFOO IHOP TRAI HTAN
LISH HOUG NOFT SEMY

Move groups of letters around to form a word. Cross off letters once used.

     __   h   o   p   e   __   __ __ __ __

        __ __   __ __ __ __

     __ __   t h o u g h t

        __ __ __   __ __ __ __

          __ __ __ __ __ __ __ .

The following words can be found in the diagram below reading forward, backward, up, down and diagonally. Find the words and circle them.

messy
jumbled
fragmented
partial
unsettled
wrong

broken
tired
awful

```
Z  G  T  X  J  A  B  Q  F  V  X  Q  L  S  P  P
W  R  V  Y  Z  G  W  H  T  W  F  O  L  X  A  F
Z  X  M  T  U  V  T  W  M  Z  R  K  P  R  D  C
F  Z  T  B  Y  T  I  V  B  B  S  T  T  G  P  E
D  E  V  E  C  H  X  X  D  R  T  I  Q  R  L  B
E  H  O  E  N  O  Y  O  N  R  A  R  W  I  S  X
T  A  Z  N  E  E  J  I  D  L  G  E  R  G  D  V
N  Y  X  L  Q  I  M  E  Y  X  R  D  L  L  P  D
E  A  Y  G  X  G  L  Z  U  H  Z  I  M  E  R  E
M  V  K  I  C  T  U  O  D  B  L  P  R  U  C  L
G  Q  R  T  T  C  F  C  I  C  B  P  Z  W  H  B
A  P  U  E  P  P  W  C  B  N  E  K  O  R  B  M
R  T  S  U  W  D  A  D  Z  S  G  A  D  O  W  U
F  N  R  X  Z  I  O  S  K  R  B  N  S  N  R  J
U  M  A  G  H  P  V  K  R  O  E  O  S  G  H  N
K  M  E  S  S  Y  O  N  O  L  F  L  K  N  A  C
```

Puzzle 6

WORKSHEET

Write a story about the day you realized you'll never feel "just right." Start the story with "I can never be perfect or feel complete again... and as a result of all this imperfection this might happen..." Write the story over and over until your anxiety drops. If it's too hard to tell the whole story, then try writing a little bit of the story-- a few sentences. Or, just keep writing troublesome words until they are not so troublesome. Repeat, repeat, repeat.

Anxiety level at start ____

Anxiety level at end ____ If your anxiety hasn't dropped, repeat this Worksheet.

Each of these Cryptograms is a message in substitution code. THE SILLY DOG might become UJD WQPPZ BVN if U is substituted for T, J for H, D for E, etc. One way to break the code is to look for repeated letters. E, T, A, O, N, R and I are the most often used letters. A single letter is usually A or I; OF, IS and IT are common 2-letter words; try THE or AND for a 3-letter group. The code is different for each Cryptogram.

1.
E
Qtqg ciahwi X šag'c hgsqdecjgs, X'z
g
gac jeuxgw̌ jwjxǧ.
n

2.
E
Dldr ptbhfť Q ňgr'p gňd ptqw, Q'e
h   a   c
fbqrf pb ab qp rbc.

3.
I   l   e
Jy J ilwul scjt xmnĺtqiulr,
tqplscjm̌v dwr ojii čwhhlm.
n   h

Below is a list of scrambled words. Unscramble all the letters to reveal the words.

Look for words that begin with "un, "in" or end with "ly" "ed" "ive."

1. ZRHDAALYHAP = _____

2. NDGRAUEZOIN = _____

3. KIWNDERL = _____

4. CNINOEIVCSLU = _____

5. UTEMN = _____

6. UINFDNHSIE = _____

7. NTSEP = _____

8. CUNOICEILSNV = _____

WORKSHEET

Use this worksheet to repeatedly write any troublesome words. Use some of your own words that you haven't seen yet in a puzzle. Fill the page with words that trigger your anxiety about never feeling "just right." Never feeling complete. Always feeling gross or "just wrong." While you're doing it if you note any anxiety say, "Good there's my anxiety. I want this so that I can practice living with it."

Anxiety level at start ____

Anxiety level at end _____

Form 5 different 5-letter words by using all the given letters and adding the letter in the Free Letter Box as often as necessary. Cross off each letter in the Letter Bank as you use it.

Free Letter	Letter Bank
e	a a b d d g m m n o r s s t t u u u v y y

1. <u>d</u> ___ ___ ___ ___

2. ___ ___ ___ ___ <u>y</u>

3. <u>m</u> ___ ___ ___ ___

4. ___ ___ ___ ___ <u>t</u>

5. ___ ___ <u>g</u> ___ ___

The spaces between the words in the following message have been eliminated and divided into pieces. Rearrange the pieces to reconstruct the messages. The dashes indicate the number of letters in each word.

SPEL DAND SWOR IMGO BEAN INGT
LTHI XIOU OMIS SNOW

— ' —   — — — — —

— —   — — — — — —
t   h   i   s
— — — —   — — — —

— — — —   — —   — — — — — —
n   o   w   .
— — —

Clue: You can probably find this kind of mistake in the book. It's clear the author isn't perfect.

Puzzle 10

WORKSHEET

Instead of telling the story, you can draw out the story. Using stick figures draw four scenes playing out your worst fear. In the first scene you realize you've made a mistake ... And then what happens next? Are you sued? Does someone die? Draw that. And then what happens? Draw that. In the final scene, draw the worst unhappy ending as a result of making a mistake. Repeat this drawing until it no longer bothers you. If it's not a mistake you fear, draw what happens if you're stuck feeling gross or "just wrong."

Anxiety level at start ____

Anxiety level at end____
If your anxiety doesn't drop, repeat this Worksheet until it does.

The following words can be found in the diagram below reading forward, backward, up, down and diagonally. Find the words and circle them.

improper	vague
shoddy	awful
deficient	unsaid
iffy	wrong
unachieved	flawed
inaccurate	partly

```
I W I F F Y E A D U A W F U L K
Z N E W X B J N U V P N Z Q X I
I I H R O R N J J Q I C Y E N U
M S H O D D Y H Z I V C J A U N
P H Q N N E S X R M A S C H N A
R A S G Y Y B F N S G C S W S C
O C J E F I J M I R U P R Y A H
P F F C X D U K T R E V B K I I
E O Z I P F V N A I Y R L H D E
R W Q Q F D E T Y W S P V F Y V
V Y W Y S I E G U U R I U L A E
Y A V G C Y N R G K I W P A L D
U M E I K H D F F Z E Y G W Y T
Y H F N Y G O U M M I E T E S M
P E I Y J U D U C G Z H G D D G
D M C Z K K N I Q P A R T L Y B
```

Puzzle 11

Each of these Cryptograms is a message in substitution code. THE SILLY DOG might become UJD WQPPZ BVN if U is substituted for T, J for H, D for E, etc. One way to break the code is to look for repeated letters. E, T, A, O, N, R and I are the most often used letters. A single letter is usually A or I; OF, IS and IT are common 2-letter words; try THE or AND for a 3-letter group. The code is different for each Cryptogram.

1. N'a jpndj ep anrrmhuu eqnr ypxc bdc
th bdznpkr dpy. (Clue: This is a great exposure exercise!)

l over nr, s over the r in eqnr

2. Km gkwe km N jwq, N bnxgj tyryw dy
kdlry krywkxy. (Clue: Mediocrity has it's benefits.)

A over Km, b over kdlry, r over tyryw, g over krywkxy

3. D'y btdab ft qths u qtf tm hqssc ol
atf mssqdab xtycqsfs. (Clue: Mediocrity has it's benefits.)

I over D'y, o over qths, a over u, l over hqssc, e over xtycqsfs

WORKSHEET

As before, using stick figures draw four scenes playing out your worst fear about not being perfect and making mistakes or feeling "just wrong" all the time. When you become desensitized to this story, draw a new story. Draw about feeling incomplete or gross and what happens if you can't get rid of these feelings.

Anxiety level at start ____

Anxiety level at end____ Keep drawing until your anxiety drops.

Don't forget to email Tammy about your Worksheets (tammy@bossitback.com) and get your secret code to unlock a hidden blog post at blog.bossitback.com. Completing the Worksheets deserves a little reward!

The below messages are in a number code based on how text messages are formed on a 'flip phone'. Each number represents one of the letters shown on the picture of the phone to the left. You must decide which one. A number is not necessarily the same letter each time.

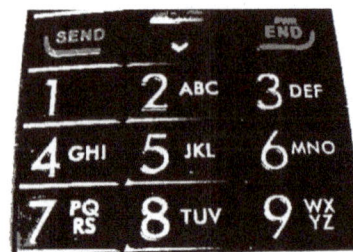

1. 43 7373328466 927 76774253 93'3 4283
66 6333 86 5683.

(Clue: Thankfully we know how to forgive and love unconditionally.)

2. 4'6 46464 86 3245 28 7373328466 27
6824 27 76774253.

(Clue: It's better to do this willingly than resist being imperfect.)

The following words can be found in the diagram below reading forward, backward, up, down and diagonally. Find the words and circle them.

disarray   tears
inexact   angry
hurried   tardy
muddled
unkept
weak

U Q T A R D Y Y I R I P V U O S
M Z A C H F E U K Y R U P T W I
Y U N K E P T J R B U H V L N F
E C G O T X I H Q V H W S E D M
W Y R W V P R L J N J E X T F K
H N Y M G Y R L B F F A Z O N D
U P J U H N H E L D C K Z B U I
R K L I T E N E R T Z L Q R X S
R R W C Q L P F V K N I R S T A
I V R V Q T D C G Y W K M B C R
E M N S D E K K A N A L D G H R
D N U P L A E M J A E F Q G L A
P D W D B R E Y O R R S B B S Y
O C D E S S J M F D B K P L K T
Q U B A C Q D Y S H W G Y N Y A
M P R P R W H A I N D K X T V I

Puzzle 14

WORKSHEET

Write a story about the day you realized you'll never be perfect ... never feel "just right." Start the story with "I can never ... as a result this might happen..." Write the story over and over until your anxiety drops. If it's too hard to tell the whole story, then try writing a little bit of the story-- a few sentences. Or, just keep writing troublesome words until they are not so troublesome. Repeat, repeat, repeat.

Anxiety level at start ____

Anxiety level at end _____

The spaces between the words in the following message has been eliminated and divided into pieces. Rearrange the pieces to reconstruct the messages. The dashes indicate the number of letters in each word.

GGED EDRA LETG OORB

L   e   t   __ __ __   __ __   __ __

b   e   __ __ __ __ __ __ __ .

The following words can be found in the diagram below reading forward, backward, up,
down and diagonally. Find the words and circle them.

unpleasant   broken
tired   tardy
awful   unmet
hurried   angry
invalid
incoherent

```
I  I  P  B  T  B  U  D  E  I  R  R  U  H  Z  Y
J  N  B  Q  O  A  T  D  I  G  A  M  B  J  B  H
Q  F  V  E  H  E  A  M  C  V  T  A  R  D  Y  T
V  R  W  A  P  T  R  O  S  A  P  I  O  O  Q  I
A  W  F  U  L  B  S  Y  H  T  L  R  K  V  S  R
H  A  W  O  E  I  X  B  H  S  X  Z  E  P  M  E
T  G  B  L  H  T  D  R  T  W  H  V  N  P  F  D
D  I  R  U  D  J  N  B  E  G  Q  J  D  S  R  W
P  Q  M  B  J  T  D  E  U  A  U  O  X  B  J  A
M  H  M  V  Y  H  Y  I  R  J  D  P  Z  N  T  N
S  E  P  H  U  C  J  E  T  E  M  N  U  V  M  G
Z  W  G  N  U  I  X  G  P  J  H  B  O  R  A  R
X  A  E  M  Z  R  F  R  V  V  Z  O  Q  X  I  Y
U  T  V  T  Q  C  H  K  L  E  Q  A  C  O  S  P
F  S  M  F  W  Y  F  O  E  X  J  Z  W  N  Z  W
F  U  Q  B  T  N  A  S  A  E  L  P  N  U  I  N
```

Puzzle 16

Each of these Cryptograms is a message in substitution code. THE SILLY DOG might become UJD WQPPZ BVN if U is substituted for T, J for H, D for E, etc. One way to break the code is to look for repeated letters. E, T, A, O, N, R and I are the most often used letters. A single letter is usually A or I; OF, IS and IT are common 2-letter words; try THE or AND for a 3-letter group. The code is different for each Cryptogram.

1. Ubyd V nbtqy lx uytodynnyn hymhcy lviba ctrib.
e   s   g   n   h
(Clue: Who cares!)

2. R'x ycruy oc ma oja jtvvrazo rubcxvaoauo vagzcu jaga.
I   o   h   t
(Clue: Who cares!!!! Whatever! So what!)

3. Iaylkfkq aynnkjx aynnkjx.
W   p   e
(Clue: Surrender and be free!)

The below messages are in a number code based on how text messages are formed on a 'flip phone'. Each number represents one of the letters shown on the picture of the phone to the left. You must decide which one. A number is not necessarily the same letter each time.

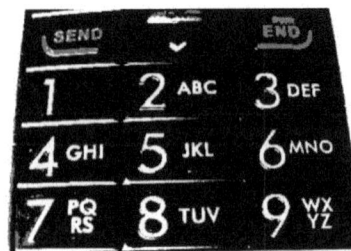

1. 4 226 63837 36 366844 86 23 7373328.
                         enough   perfect

    (Clue: It's the human factor.)

2. 4'6 46464 86 5673 2 568 63 75337 29
    going   sleep

    668 3335464 26675383.

    (Clue: The day will be harder but oh well.)

Puzzle 18

WORKSHEET

Your Choice: Either write troublesome words, or write a "once upon a time" story about waking up with that "just wrong" or gross feeling and being stuck with the discomfort and uncertainty. If you're not feeling much anxiety, make sure you're not avoiding any words or stories.

Anxiety level at start ____

Anxiety level at end _____

Form 5 different 5-letter words by using all the given letters and adding the letter in the Free Letter Box as often as necessary. Cross off each letter in the Letter Bank as you use it.

Free Letter	Letter Bank
a	d e e f g l m n n o r r r s t t t u u w w y

1. a ___ ___ ___ ___

2. ___ ___ ___ ___ g ___

3. t ___ ___ ___ ___

4. ___ ___ ___ s ___

5. u ___ ___ ___ ___

To solve this puzzle, fill in the blanks below with the correct missing letter and then transfer the letter to the corresponding numbered square in the diagram below. Be careful! The puzzle is not as simple as it may first appear!

1.	2.	3.	4.	5.	6.	7.	8.	9.	10.

1. a w f _ l

2. b r o k e _

3. u n t _ u e

4. t _ a r s

5. f _ a w e d

6. t i r _ d

7. w e _ k

8. u n _ a i d

9. u n k _ p t

10. s h o _ d y

Puzzle 20

WORKSHEET

Using stick figures draw four scenes playing out your worst fear about not being perfect and making mistakes or feeling "just wrong" all the time. When you become desensitized to this story, draw a new story. Draw about feeling incomplete or gross and what happens if you can't get rid of these feelings. Repeat this until you're bored drawing it. The whole point of repeating an exposure over and over is to get bored!

Anxiety level at start _____

Anxiety level at end _____

The following words can be found in the diagram below reading forward, backward, up, down and diagonally. Find the words and circle them.

consumed   unkept
unsettled   messy
shoddy   flawed
unfinished   late
unresolved
weak

B U H O U U N F I N I S H E D P

U T N E M A X R M G H O Q W M T

N U Z R S B U Y D U M Q S R R Z

K G M W E A K P Z Q B A O T N V

E A B M X S O G R O Y S I X W C

P K N V B E O V I R K I H M I W

T F W S G Y E L D N K V B J O K

G K N R X I T D V C D B T O J B

A S Y G O Q M N E E U P B F K C

M O Y M V J Y A M L D H I F J M

E H D B Q F D B I E T I X U U L

S F L A W E D P K L A T E M V V

S O J T B F O D B R K K E X U W

Y E Y Y V E H Z D I I B D S C M

T M Y O H N S Y B O D F Q V N Q

A S K X X C O N S U M E D J V U

Puzzle 21

Below is a list of scrambled words. Unscramble all the letters to reveal the words.
(Clue: Look for word endings like "ion" "ed" "ive")

1. SSONIIOM =
   _____

2. DEATXSUHE =
   _____

3. DAZYLHAHRAP =
   _____

4. ZZYTI =
   _____

5. OKBREN =
   _____

6. SYARDRAI =
   _____

7. RRHDUEI =
   _____

8. EERPTIEIVT =
   _____

Puzzle 22

WORKSHEET

Write a story about the day you realized you'll never obtain perfection... Start the story with "I can never feel "just right" about ... and as a result this might happen..." If your anxiety is remains high, consider reading your story out loud, using an accent.

Anxiety level at start ____

Anxiety level at end _____

Place two letters on the dashes to complete a word on the left and to begin another word on the right. For example, SE in between PLEA and VEN would complete PLEASE and begin SEVEN.

1. d e s p e r a _ _ a r s

2. u n w h o l e s o _ _ s s y

3. u n c e r t a _ _ e p t

4. o v e r r _ _ m e t

5. p l _ _ e l e s s

Rearrange and distribute the five letters accompanying each row so
that you form a larger common word.

1. m e r e :   i __ p __ __ c i s __

2. d e e p :   u n __ __ r f o r m __ __

3. f i r e :   __ m p __ __ __ e c t

4. b l u e :   __ n __ a __ a n c __ d

5. f i v e :   d __ __ e c t __ __ e

WORKSHEET

Your Method of Choice: Either write troublesome words, write a never feeling "just right" story, or use stick figures to draw out four horror scenes about being imperfect or grossed out... Of the three methods are you choosing the easiest all the time? Work your way up to the hardest method. It's important to build momentum.
Remember what you're fighting for.

Anxiety level at start _____

Anxiety level at end _____

Insert a different letter of the alphabet into each of the 26 empty boxes to form words reading across. The letter you insert may be at the beginning, the end or the middle of the word. Each letter of the alphabet will be used only once. Cross off each letter in the list as you use it. All the letters in each row are not necessarily used in forming the word.

Example: In the first row, we have inserted the letter Z to form the word TIZZY

A B C D E F G H I J K L M N O P Q R S T U V W X Y Z̶

U	F	Y	T	I	Z	**Z**	Y	A	L	T	E	X
F	L	U	S	T	E		E	D	G	I	J	H
C	E	X	H	A	U		T	E	D	E	E	X
I	N	T	E	R	R		P	T	B	W	G	G
A	C	U	N	K	E		T	O	S	J	V	O
E	L	F	U	N	F		N	I	S	H	E	D
I	Q	V	A	A	N		R	Y	H	H	P	Q
U	T	K	H	A	L		W	A	Y	J	P	X
C	D	I	N	C	O		P	L	E	T	E	K
V	T	W	R	I	N		L	E	D	B	P	E
H	H	R	E	P	E		I	T	I	V	E	H
I	M	P	R	O	P		R	V	M	E	D	N
L	E	P	A	R	T		Y	B	T	V	W	U
W	T	C	S	G	H		U	M	B	L	E	D
M	U	D	D	L	E		T	L	E	S	I	X
T	O	Y	E	Y	E		D	L	E	S	S	Y
R	R	M	I	M	B		L	A	N	C	E	D
Y	Q	L	Q	Z	A		F	U	L	G	E	C
U	Z	D	E	F	E		T	I	V	E	K	P
E	J	I	I	N	E		A	C	T	M	S	Q
C	I	N	A	D	E		U	A	T	E	X	E
L	O	L	K	Z	A		U	R	R	I	E	D
U	E	L	Y	I	N		A	L	I	D	N	X
O	S	C	R	A	M		L	E	D	J	D	Y
F	D	J	I	N	C		R	R	E	C	T	L
P	W	A	N	N	O		E	D	U	M	E	B

Puzzle 25

WORKSHEET

If you've gotten used to the words and images associated with being imperfect, it's time to take bigger steps. Are there any people, places or things you've been avoiding because of your imperfections? Make a list of them. If you were to stop avoiding, rate them in terms of most anxiety- provoking to least. Starting with the least anxiety- provoking trigger, it's time to stop avoiding and live your life. Begin your gradual mission to face whatever you're avoiding. It might be hard. But, it's your path to freedom.

Anxiety level at start ____

Anxiety level at end _____

WORKSHEET

Use this page to practice your Boss it Back voice.

OCD says: Get this to be perfect. You can't afford a mistake.
Boss it Back: If I make a mistake, so be it.

OCD says: If you don't get this right, it's going to bother you all day and night.
Boss it Back: If I feel impending doom for days on end, so be it.

OCD says: You're going to look foolish if you don't think of something intelligent to say right now.
Boss it Back: I hope I lose my train of thought! We need a good laugh!

OCD says: People will think badly of you if you mess up. *Boss it Back: Yes, I'll be remembered for all my imperfections.*

OCD says: It's not germy, it's just gross. You'll feel gross all day if you don't fix it.
Boss it Back: I'm not going to fix it. I'm just going to let the anxiety exist while I go on about normal living.

OCD says: You better get more clarification or you'll mess this up.
You agree: True, I might mess up. But then again, I might not. Time will tell.

OCD says: What will people think if they see you like this?
You agree: Maybe they'll think I'm a farce. Time will tell.

In Summary

Tips to Remember

❖ Repetition breeds boredom.

❖ Confront your fear repeatedly and you will get bored.

❖ Avoidance breeds anxiety.

❖ Experience anxiety with curiosity.

❖ Face your fears and feel the anxiety.

❖ Agree with OCD, don't argue with it.

❖ Talk to OCD as if feeling "just wrong" doesn't matter to you.

❖ Repeatedly confront trigger words, stories and drawings.

❖ Make sure you repeatedly do it.

❖ When you become desensitized to words move on to real situations.

❖ If you only confront a feared situation sporadically, it'll likely be traumatic.

❖ Confront your fears repeatedly. And accelerate. Build momentum.

FINAL WORDS

About the Author

o Tammy LaBrake, is a licensed Clinical Social Worker (LCSW) and founder of a private practice in New York known as, Boss It Back® which is dedicated to the treatment of OCD.

o As an unorthodox thinker, she values cutting edge developments and enjoys using creativity in her practice.

o Tammy agrees with the evidence-based power of Exposure & Response (ERP) therapy in the treatment of OCD. It's important to address OCD as soon as possible and so she created a series of OCD puzzle books to make ERP exercises readily available.

o Tammy is a member of the International OCD Foundation and is a graduate of the Foundation's Behavior Training Therapy Institute.

o She is the author of other publications such as the innovative OCD Coloring Book.

o For more ideas on ERP, visit blog.bossitback.com and search Exposure & Response Prevention.

o If you would like to receive tips on a regular basis, please join Tammy's free email list at: OCDstrategies.com

o You can also follow Tammy on Twitter at: @tjlabrake or Facebook (Search: Free Your Life. Free Your Mind. Defy OCD.)

o And if you are interested in learning more about other publications by Tammy, please visit: Tammy's Author Page on Amazon.

Best wishes in your Boss it Back endeavors! You're stronger than you know!

ANSWER KEY

From Puzzle 2

It is what it is and I accept this feeling of doom.

I hope I lose my train of thought and look foolish.

People will remember me for my imperfections.

Puzzle 3

I'm going to make this mistake and allow the anxiety to overwhelm me.

A perfection mindset fails.

A growth mindset learns.

Puzzle 4

¹u	²s	³e	⁴l	⁵e	⁶s	⁷s

1. f a <u>u</u> l t y

2. t e a r <u>s</u>

3. w <u>e</u> a k

4. a w f u <u>l</u>

5. m <u>e</u> s s y

6. c h a o <u>s</u>

7. <u>s</u> l o w

Puzzle 5

i   h o p e   i   l o s e

m y   t r a i n

o f   t h o u g h t

a n d   l o o k

f o o l i s h

ANSWER KEY

Puzzle 7

Even though I don't understand, I'm not asking again.

Even though I can't ace this, I'm going to do it now.

If I leave this unresolved, something bad will happen.

Puzzle 8

1. ZRHDAALYHAP = **HAPHAZARDLY**

2. NDGRAUEZOIN = **UNORGANIZED**

3. KIWNDERL = **WRINKLED**

4. CNINOEIVCSLU = **INCONCLUSIVE**

5. UTEMN = **UNMET**

6. UINFDNHSIE = **UNFINISHED**

7. NTSEP = **SPENT**

8. CUNOICEILSNV = **INCONCLUSIVE**

Puzzle 9

1. d o u b t
2. t a r d y
3. m e s s y
4. u n m e t
5. v a g u e

Puzzle 10

i'm going
to misspell
this word
and be anxious
now.

ANSWER KEY

Puzzle 12

I'm going to misspell this word and be anxious now.

As hard as I try, I might never be above average.

I'm going to lose a lot of sleep by not feeling complete.

Puzzle 13

If perfection was possible we'd have no need to love.

I'm going to fail at perfection as much as possible.

Puzzle 15

Let go or be dragged

Puzzle 17

When I share my weaknesses people might laugh.

I'm going to be the happiest incompetent person here.

Whatever happens happens.

ANSWER KEY

Puzzle 18

I can never do enough to be perfect.

I'm going to lose a lot of sleep by not feeling complete.

Puzzle 19

1. awful
2. wrong
3. tardy
4. tears
5. unmet

Puzzle 20

u	n	r	e	l	e	a	s	e	d

1. a w f <u>u</u> l
2. b r o k e <u>n</u>
3. u n t <u>r</u> u e
4. t <u>e</u> a r s
5. f <u>l</u> a w e d
6. t i r <u>e</u> d
7. w e <u>a</u> k
8. u n <u>s</u> a i d
9. u n k <u>e</u> p t
10. s h o <u>d</u> d y

Puzzle 22

1. SSONIIOM = **OMISSION**
2. DEATXSUHE = **EXHAUSTED**
3. DAZYLHAHRAP = **HAPHAZARDLY**
4. ZZYTI = **TIZZY**
5. OKBREN = **BROKEN**
6. SYARDRAI = **DISARRAY**
7. RRHDUEI = **HURRIED**
8. EERPTIEIVT = **REPETITIVE**

ANSWER KEY

Puzzle 23

1. d e s p e r a <u>t</u> <u>e</u> a r s

2. u n w h o l e s o m <u>e</u> s s y

3. u n c e r t a <u>i</u> <u>n</u> e p t

4. o v e r r u <u>n</u> m e t

5. p l u <u>s</u> <u>e</u> l e s s

Puzzle 24

1. mere: i <u>m</u> p <u>r</u> e c i s <u>e</u>

2. deep: u n p <u>e</u> r f o r m <u>e</u> d

3. fire: <u>i</u> m p <u>e</u> r <u>f</u> e c t

4. blue: <u>u</u> <u>n</u> b <u>a</u> l a n c <u>e</u> d

5. five: d <u>e</u> f e c t <u>i</u> <u>v</u> e

Puzzle 25

U	F	Y	T	I	Z	**Z**	Y	A	L	T	E	X
F	L	U	S	T	E	R	E	D	G	I	J	H
C	E	X	H	A	U	S	T	E	D	E	E	X
I	N	T	E	R	R	U	P	T	B	W	G	G
A	C	U	N	K	E	P	T	O	S	J	V	O
E	L	F	U	N	F	I	N	I	S	H	E	D
I	Q	V	A	A	N	G	R	Y	H	H	P	Q
U	T	K	H	A	L	F	W	A	Y	J	P	X
C	D	I	N	C	O	M	P	L	E	T	E	K
V	T	W	R	I	N	K	L	E	D	B	P	E
H	H	R	E	P	E	T	I	T	I	V	E	H
I	M	P	R	O	P	E	R	V	M	E	D	N
L	E	P	A	R	T	L	Y	B	T	V	W	U
W	T	C	S	G	H	J	U	M	B	L	E	D
M	U	D	D	L	E	D	T	L	E	S	I	X
T	O	Y	E	Y	E	N	D	L	E	S	S	Y
R	R	M	I	M	B	A	L	A	N	C	E	D
Y	Q	L	Q	Z	A	W	F	U	L	G	E	C
U	Z	D	E	F	E	C	T	I	V	E	K	P
E	J	I	I	N	E	X	A	C	T	M	S	Q
C	I	N	A	D	E	Q	U	A	T	E	X	E
L	O	L	K	Z	A	H	U	R	R	I	E	D
U	E	L	Y	I	N	V	A	L	I	D	N	X
O	S	C	R	A	M	B	L	E	D	J	D	Y
F	D	J	I	N	C	O	R	R	E	C	T	L
P	W	A	N	N	O	Y	E	D	U	M	E	B